CARNIVORE DIET FOR SENIORS

The Essential Guide And Secrets To Lose Weight, Revitalize Health And Vitality With Meat-Based Recipes

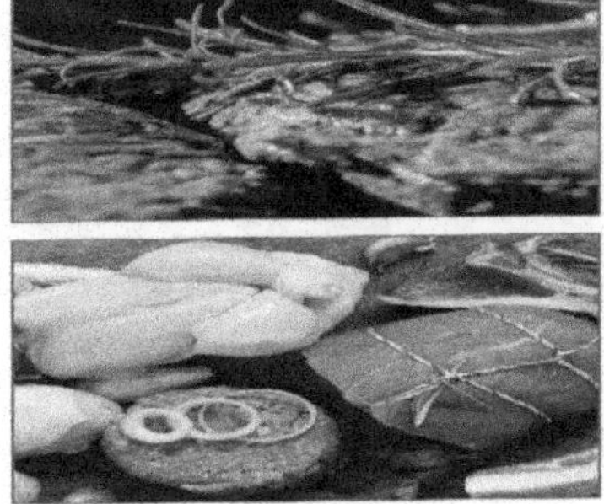

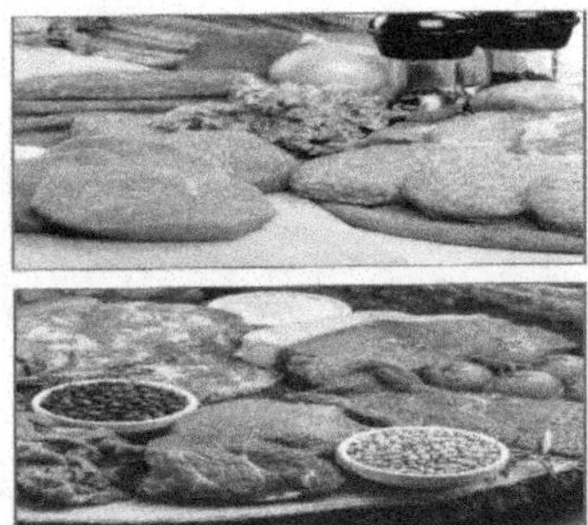

LINDA DONLEY

TABLE OF CONTENTS

TABLE OF CONTENTS 2

INTRODUCTION 6

CHAPTER ONE.. 12

    Understanding the Carnivore Diet................................ 12

    The Carnivore Diet's Historical Roots and Evolution........... 12

    Benefits of the Carnivore Diet 13

    Controversies Surrounding the Carnivore Diet.................... 14

    Navigating the Carnivore Landscape 14

CHAPTER TWO.. 16

    Nurturing Vitality in the Golden Years......................... 16

    Common Dietary Challenges for Older Adults..................... 18

CHAPTER THREE 20

    Basics of the Carnivore Diet 20

    What is the Carnivore Diet?.................................... 20

    Principles of the Carnivore Diet............................... 21

    Guidelines for a Carnivorous Expedition:....................... 23

    Navigating the Carnivorous Wilderness 25

CHAPTER FOUR 26

    The Comprehensive Health Benefits of the Carnivore Diet for Seniors... 26

CHAPTER FIVE 30

    Navigating the Carnivore Journey 30

Transitioning to a Carnivore Diet 30

CHAPTER SIX 34

Building a Balanced Carnivore Plate for Optimal Health 34

CHAPTER SEVEN 40

Recipes 40

10 Irresistible Carnivore Breakfast Recipes for Seniors 40

Classic Bacon and Eggs 40

Smoked Salmon Roll-ups 41

Egg and Sausage Muffins 41

Steak and Avocado Salad 42

Egg and Cheese Breakfast Casserole 42

Chicken Liver Pâté 43

Sausage and Egg Breakfast Skillet 43

Baked Ham and Cheese Omelet 44

Ground Beef Breakfast Bowl 44

Turkey and Cheese Roll-ups 45

10 Carnivore Diet Lunch Recipes Tailored for Seniors 46

Recipe 1: Chicken Caesar Salad 46

Recipe 2: Egg Salad Lettuce Wraps 47

Recipe 3: Tuna Avocado Boats 48

Recipe 4: Beef and Spinach Omelet 48

Recipe 5: Lamb Kebabs with Mint Yogurt Sauce 49

Recipe 6: Bacon-wrapped Asparagus Bundles 50

Recipe 7: Turkey and Cheese Roll-ups 50

Recipe 8: Pork Carnitas Lettuce Wraps 51

Recipe 9: Grilled Sardines with Lemon 52

Recipe 10: Salmon Patties 52

10 Satisfying Carnivore Diet Dinner Recipes 53

Recipe 1: Ribeye Steak with Garlic Butter 54

Recipe 2: Chicken Thighs with Lemon and Herbs 55

Recipe 3: Seared Scallops with Garlic Ghee 55

Recipe 4: Pork Ribs with Dry Rub 56

Recipe 5: Lamb Shank Stew 57

Recipe 6: Grilled Swordfish Steaks 57

Recipe 7: Ground Beef and Eggplant Casserole 58

Recipe 8: Turkey Bacon-wrapped Brussels Sprouts 59

Recipe 9: Bison Burger Lettuce Wraps 60

Recipe 10: Salmon and Avocado Salad 60

10 Carnivore Diet Seafood Recipes for Seniors 61

Recipe 1: Grilled Lemon Garlic Shrimp 62

Recipe 2: Baked Lemon Dill Salmon 62

Recipe 3: Garlic Butter Lobster Tails 63

Recipe 4: Tuna Steak with Sesame Crust 64

Recipe 5: Coconut Lime Shrimp Skewers 65

Recipe 6: Scallops with Bacon and Rosemary 65

Recipe 7: Lemon Butter Cod Fish 66

Recipe 8: Garlic Herb Grilled Squid 67

Recipe 9: Cajun Shrimp and Sausage Skillet 68

Recipe 10: Crab Stuffed Avocado 68

10 Carnivore Diet Snack Recipes for Seniors 70

Recipe 1: Deviled Eggs with Bacon 70

Recipe 2: Parmesan Crisps 71

Recipe 3: Beef Jerky 72

Recipe 4: Chicken Liver Pops 72

Recipe 5: Smoked Salmon Roll-ups 73

Recipe 6: Sardine Stuffed Avocado 73

Recipe 7: Cheese and Pepperoni Bites 74

Recipe 8: Ham and Cream Cheese Rolls 74

Recipe 9: Bacon-wrapped Shrimp 75

Recipe 10: Prosciutto-wrapped Asparagus 75

CHAPTER EIGHT 78

28-day meal plan 78

CONCLUSION 88

Embracing Vitality in the Golden Years with the Carnivore Diet 88

Highlights from Our Culinary Expedition 88

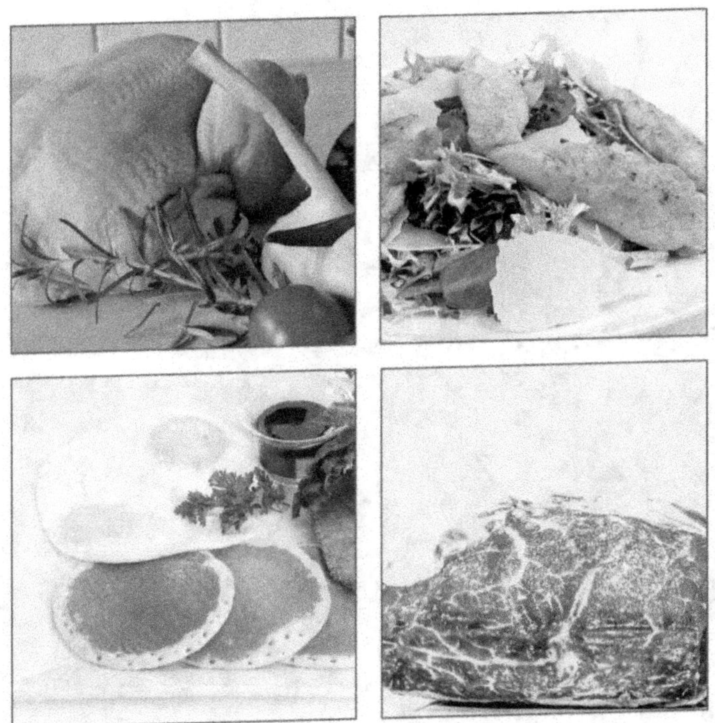

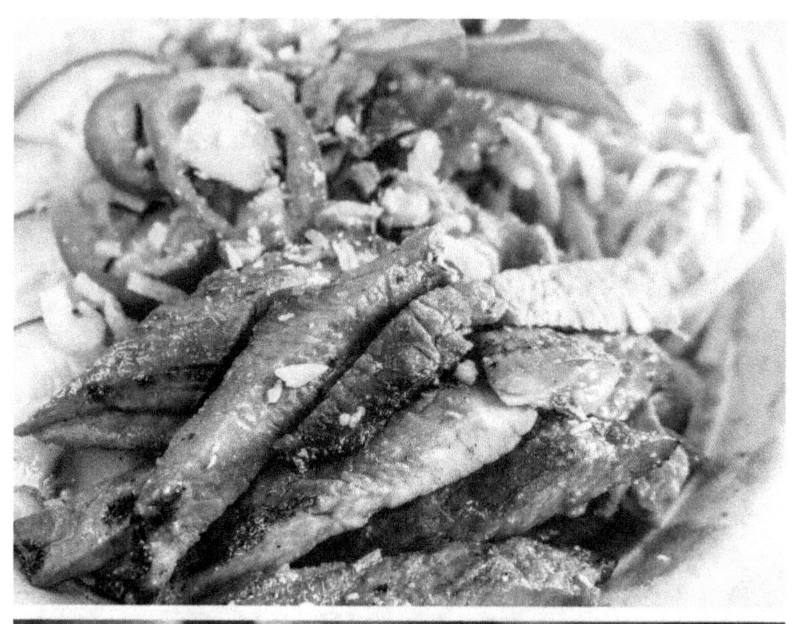

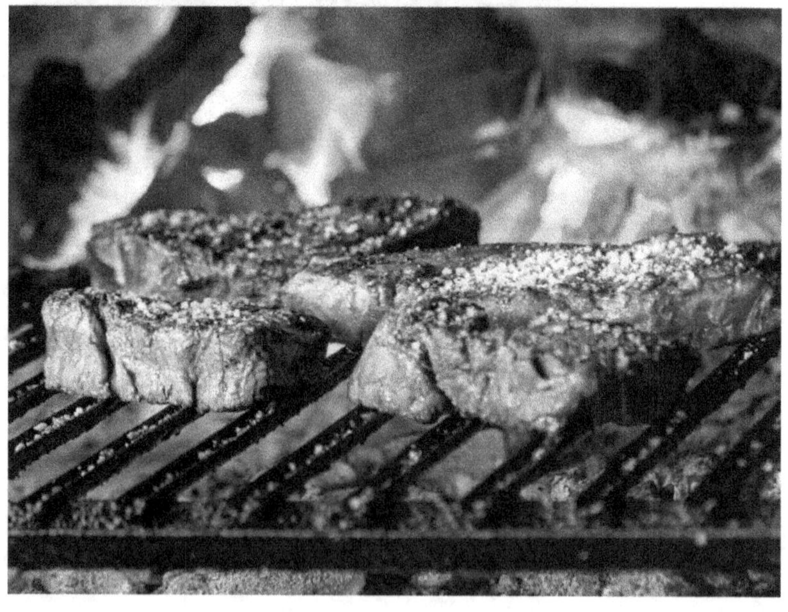

In the domain of health, my adventure with the Carnivore Diet for Seniors wasn't simply a dietary transition; it was a metamorphosis—an expedition from skepticism to a symphony of vigor that rang through the golden years.

The experience started with the flip of the book's first page when misgivings loomed huge. "Can an all-meat diet truly be the key to unlocking renewed energy and well-being?" I pondered. Little did I realize that this investigation would become a transformational adventure, challenging conventional beliefs and altering the story of aging.

The first chapter, "Understanding Senior Nutrition," established the scene, revealing the nuances of the specialized dietary demands that characterize the golden years. As the pages rolled, I found myself nodding in accord, recognizing the subtle changes in my own body and the urge for a nutritional strategy that matched the symphony of my age.

Then came the revelation—the "Basics of the Carnivore Diet." The carnivorous forest beckoned, and I hesitated at the threshold. Yet, with every piece of pan-seared fish and every delectable grilled ribeye, I found a universe of sensations that defied expectations. The ideas of the diet—minimalism, quality above quantity, and a celebration of animal elegance—became the guiding lights of my culinary voyage.

As the chapters unfolded, the health advantages presented themselves like buried jewels. Improved joint health enabled me to dance through the years, while increased cognitive function became the key to opening the door to mental clarity. The Carnivore Diet wasn't simply a food option; it was a compass pointing toward a world of well-being that I hadn't considered attainable.

Meal planning and cooking were the center of my trip. The sizzle of lamb chops with mint pesto, the succulence of bacon-wrapped asparagus bundles—each dish was a celebration of sustenance, a smorgasbord of sensations expertly prepared for the seasoned palette. My kitchen changed into a stage, where the Carnivore Diet meals stole the limelight, and I became the chef of my own health story.

Addressing fears and misunderstandings became a time of empowerment. Armed with information, I challenged critics and questioned the misconceptions surrounding the Carnivore Diet. The issues that had loomed huge now felt like faraway shadows, and I stood in the brightness of educated decision-making.

But the actual crescendo of my trip reverberated in the success stories and testimonials—the real-life experiences that formed an image of renewed energy, vibrancy, and pleasure. Seniors like myself challenged prejudices, becoming real evidence that the Carnivore Diet wasn't just a book title; it was a guide to a chapter of life full of vigor.

As I near the finish of my Carnivore Diet for Seniors trip, I look back at the skeptic I once was and wonder at the turnaround. What began as a culinary investigation became a passport to energy, a monument to the reality that health recognizes no age restrictions.

Today, I stand not only as a reader but as a protagonist in my own success story—a narrative of a carnivorous adventure that converted doubt into vigor, and each chapter unfurled with the promise that the best is yet to come in the golden years. The Carnivore Diet for Seniors wasn't just a book; it was the map that took me toward a path of health, and the pages of my life continue to spin with increased vitality, resilience, and the delight of relishing every moment.

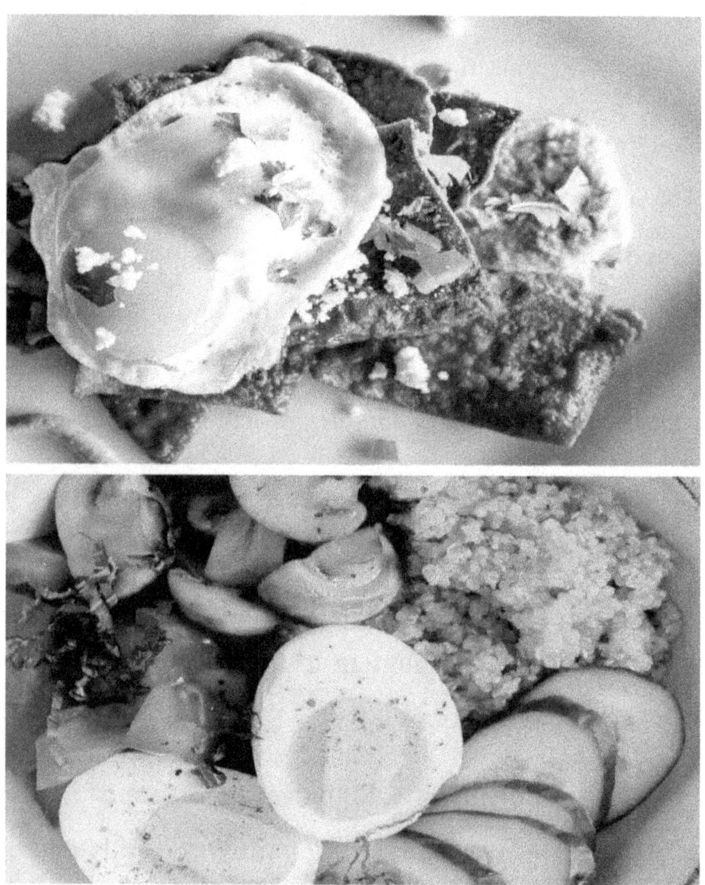

CHAPTER ONE

Understanding the Carnivore Diet

In the enormous field of nutritional options, the Carnivore Diet stands out as an intriguing outlier. Rooted in the primitive act of ingesting animal food solely, it marks a deviation from mainstream dietary thinking. To grasp this nutritional strategy, one needs to go into its historical origins, evolutionary background, and the intricate interplay of advantages and concerns that surround it.

The Carnivore Diet's Historical Roots and Evolution

The roots of the Carnivore Diet were sowed in our evolutionary history when early humans, as hunter-gatherers, depended primarily on animal sources for nutrition. As people settled and agriculture took the role, the human diet varied. However, proponents of the Carnivore Diet say that our genetic composition preserves an ancient preference for animal-derived nutrients.

The present revival of the Carnivore Diet may be linked back to the studies of scholars like Dr. Vilhjalmur Stefansson in the early 20th century and, more recently, prominent personalities like Dr. Shawn Baker. This diet concentrates emphasis on animal proteins and fats while rejecting plant-based meals, claiming to promote a return to the nutritional fundamentals of our species.

Benefits of the Carnivore Diet

The Carnivore Diet has attracted attention for its supposed advantages, both anecdotal and, to some degree, validated by developing scientific investigations. Advocates believe that by avoiding plant-based meals, people may have improved digestion, greater mental clarity, higher energy levels, and better management of certain health ailments, including autoimmune illnesses and metabolic difficulties.

Some proponents argue that the Carnivore Diet may be a strong tool for weight control, noting the satiating quality of animal fats and proteins, which may naturally lead to lower calorie consumption.

Controversies Surrounding the Carnivore Diet

While the Carnivore Diet has its enthusiastic proponents, it is not without its fair share of controversy. Critics say that the removal of plant-based meals may lead to nutritional inadequacies, notably in vital vitamins, minerals, and fiber. The long-term health ramifications of such a limited diet remain a matter of controversy, and vigilance is advised.

Regarding the environmental consequences of a diet highly dependent on animal husbandry have spurred ethical arguments. Balancing the possible health advantages with ethical and environmental issues adds a dimension of complexity to the Carnivore Diet argument.

Navigating the Carnivore Landscape

Understanding the Carnivore Diet involves a comprehensive assessment of its historical origins, evolutionary context, and the interplay of advantages and conflicts. As people negotiate their dietary options, it is necessary to approach the Carnivore Diet with an educated perspective, noting both its potential benefits and the need for careful assessment of its limits and ethical implications. In the expanding tapestry of nutritional research, the Carnivore Diet remains a riveting chapter, challenging us to question, learn, and make choices that match with our health, beliefs, and the complicated interconnectedness of our world.

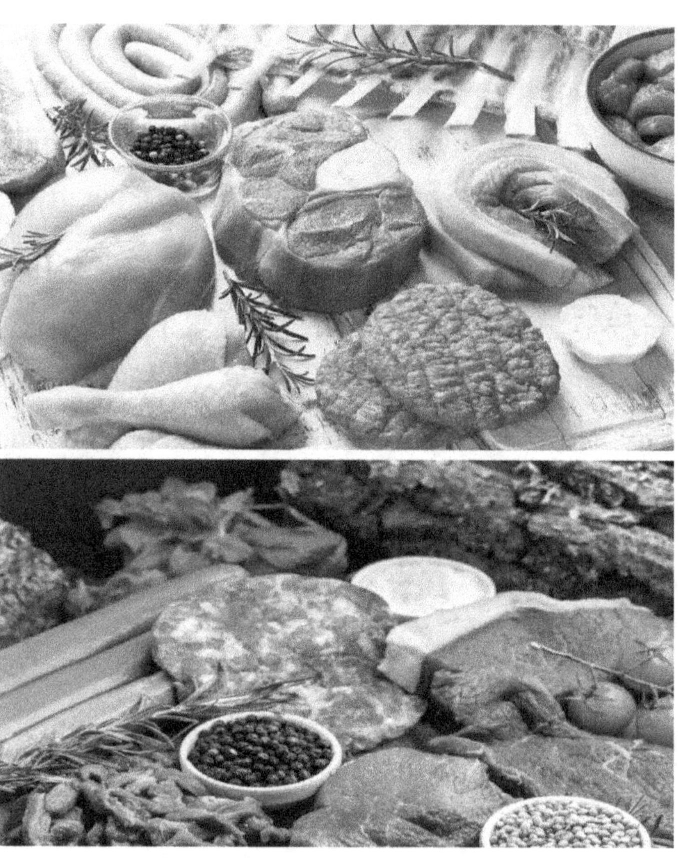

CHAPTER TWO

Nurturing Vitality in the Golden Years

As we elegantly stroll into the golden years, our bodies experience a series of changes that necessitate a more sophisticated approach to diet. The particular nutritional demands of seniors originate from a mix of variables, including changes in metabolism, diminished muscle mass, changed nutrient absorption, and the prevalence of chronic health disorders. Recognizing and fulfilling these individual needs is crucial for supporting maximum health and vigor in this beloved chapter of life.

1. Adequate Protein Intake: Seniors typically endure a loss in muscle mass and strength, a disease known as sarcopenia. To offset this, a larger intake of high-quality protein becomes important. Protein-rich meals, such as lean meats, fish, eggs, and dairy, may play a crucial role in preserving muscle mass and supporting general well-being.

2. Calcium and Vitamin D for Bone Health: Aging is accompanied by an increased risk of osteoporosis and fractures. Ensuring a sufficient diet of calcium and vitamin D is crucial for maintaining bone density and minimizing the probability of fractures. Dairy products, leafy greens, and sunshine exposure are good providers of these vital nutrients.

3. Fiber for Digestive Health: Constipation becomes more widespread with age owing to changes in the digestive tract. A diet high in fiber from whole grains, fruits, and vegetables helps regulate bowel motions and maintains a healthy digestive system.

4. Hydration: The sense of thirst tends to lessen with age, leaving seniors more prone to dehydration. Proper hydration is critical for sustaining cognitive function, renal health, and overall vigor. Encouraging the intake of water and hydrating meals is vital.

Common Dietary Challenges for Older Adults

Navigating the culinary environment in older years frequently comes with its set of obstacles, needing a strategic strategy to overcome roadblocks and maintain a well-balanced diet.

1. hunger Changes: Aging may change taste buds and reduce the sense of smell, altering hunger. Seniors may find some meals less appetizing, resulting in lower food consumption. Experimenting with tastes, and textures, and adopting nutrient-dense alternatives may help address these changes.

2. Limited Chewing Ability: Dental disorders or the loss of teeth may make chewing difficult for elders. This may restrict their options to softer foods, thereby impacting the diversity and nutritional content of their diet. Including nutrient-rich, readily chewable choices may give a solution.

3. Medication Interactions: Some drugs may impair food absorption or appetite. Seniors typically suffer from managing many medicines and need tight cooperation between healthcare practitioners and nutritionists to develop meals that complement medical treatments.

4. Social Isolation and Mental Health: Loneliness or social isolation may alter appetite and nutritional habits. Creating chances for shared meals, participating in social activities, and maintaining a good dining atmosphere may significantly improve senior nutrition.

In addressing the particular nutritional demands and problems of seniors, we pave the way for a dietary strategy that not only nourishes the body but also promotes the overall quality of life in this magnificent period of the human journey.

CHAPTER THREE

Basics of the Carnivore Diet

The Carnivore Diet, an increasingly popular nutritional strategy, stands as a compelling departure from the standard understanding of nutrition. Rooted on the idea that our evolutionary past as hunters and gatherers predisposes us to flourish on an animal-centric diet, the Carnivore Diet is a journey into simplicity, stressing the sole intake of animal products. In this research, we dig into the key concepts of the Carnivore Diet, unraveling its principles and standards that urge fans to go on a carnivorous voyage.

What is the Carnivore Diet?

At its foundation, the Carnivore Diet is a dietary regimen that emphasizes animal-derived meals while excluding plant-based ones. Enthusiasts of this method, commonly referred to as "carnivores," accept a meal dominated by meat, fish, eggs, and certain dairy products. The guiding concept is built on the notion that the human body is biologically designed to acquire the best nourishment from animal sources, matching the eating patterns of our ancient predecessors.

While the thought of an all-meat diet may first raise eyebrows, proponents believe that it delivers a plethora of health advantages, ranging from better metabolic health and weight control to greater mental clarity and energy levels. The Carnivore Diet believes that by excluding plant-based meals, consumers may eliminate possible irritants, allergies, and anti-nutrients, leading to a more basic and digestible approach to nutrition.

Principles of the Carnivore Diet

1. Animal Products as the Foundation: The cornerstone of the Carnivore Diet rests in emphasizing animal products as the major source of nourishment. This covers a range of meats such as cattle, chicken, lamb, and hog, along with fish and seafood. The focus is on ingesting both muscle meats and organ meats to provide a broad range of critical nutrients.

2. Elimination of Plant-Based Foods: A distinguishing aspect of the Carnivore Diet is the absence of plant-based foods, including fruits, vegetables, grains, legumes, and nuts. This purposeful absence derives from the assumption that certain chemicals contained in plants, such as lectins and oxalates, may cause problems with digestion and general health. By eliminating these potential irritants, proponents believe that the body can better absorb and use nutrients from animal sources.

3. Embracing Animal Fats: Contrary to standard nutritional recommendations, the Carnivore Diet puts a priority on animal fats. Saturated fats from sources like beef, pigs, and eggs are not only acceptable but recommended. Proponents say that these fats are needed for hormone synthesis, cognitive function, and general cellular health. The diet embraces the satiating characteristic of fats, giving a sensation of fullness and contentment.

4. Minimalism in Food Preparation: The Carnivore Diet frequently employs a minimalist approach to meal preparation. While others may opt to enjoy meats in different ways, such as grilled, roasted, or seared, the accent remains on simplicity. The lack of sophisticated recipes or intricate cooking techniques coincides with the primitive essence of the diet, stressing the beauty of pure animal meals.

Guidelines for a Carnivorous Expedition:

1. Quality Matters: When going on the Carnivore Diet, emphasizing the quality of animal products becomes crucial. Opting for grass-fed and pasture-raised meats, free-range poultry, and wild-caught fish guarantees a richer nutritious profile, including omega-3 fatty acids and antioxidants. Selecting organically produced animal products further lowers possible exposure to pesticides and hormones.

2. Listen to Your Body: Individual reactions to the Carnivore Diet might vary, and sensitivity to one's body is crucial. Some may find success with a rigorous all-meat strategy, while others may benefit from modest changes, such as integrating dairy or eggs. Regular self-assessment, along with modifications based on personal health indicators and well-being, enables people to personalize their diet according to their requirements.

3. Adequate Hydration: While the Carnivore Diet predominantly concentrates on animal products, water remains an important part of general wellness. Water is vital for digestion, renal function, and maintaining electrolyte balance. Ensuring an appropriate intake of water is crucial, particularly considering the lack of hydrating fruits and vegetables in the diet.

4. *Electrolyte Management:* As the Carnivore Diet restricts the consumption of plant foods, which are generally high in potassium and magnesium, humans must pay attention to electrolyte balance. Incorporating salt, magnesium supplements, and potassium-rich foods like avocados or mushrooms may help avoid electrolyte imbalances and related symptoms like muscular cramps.

5. *Monitoring Nutrient Intake:* While animal products provide a vast variety of nutrients, monitoring specific micronutrients, such as vitamin C and fiber, becomes vital. While proponents say that the body's needs for certain elements are reduced on a Carnivore Diet, it is essential to stay watchful and, if required, integrate supplements or carefully selected animal products to treat possible shortfalls.

Navigating the Carnivorous Wilderness

The Carnivore Diet, with its dramatic departure from standard dietary norms, welcomes folks into a carnivorous wilderness where the concepts of simplicity and animal-centric nutrition rule supreme. As fans begin on this culinary voyage, knowing the key ideas of the Carnivore Diet and following careful standards become the compass and chart for navigating the meaty landscape. Just as every ecosystem has its laws and rhythms, the Carnivore Diet delivers a unique symphony of animal beauty, encouraging people to investigate, adapt, and harmonize with the primordial notes of this eating choice. Whether considered a radical departure or a return to ancestral origins, the Carnivore Diet is a gastronomic experience that ignites curiosity, challenges norms, and, for some, opens the door to a fresh chapter of personal well-being and nutritional research.

CHAPTER FOUR

The Comprehensive Health Benefits of the Carnivore Diet for Seniors

As people age, prioritizing health becomes more crucial, and dietary choices play a critical part in determining overall well-being. One dietary strategy garnering attention for its possible health advantages, especially for seniors, is the carnivore diet. In this article, we will discuss three essential characteristics of the carnivorous diet that lead to greater health for seniors: increased joint health, superior cognitive performance, and successful treatment of chronic illnesses.

Improved Joint Health: Seniors commonly battle with joint concerns such as arthritis, osteoporosis, and ordinary wear and tear from a lifetime of activity. The carnivore diet, concentrated upon animal products, maybe a game-changer in enhancing joint health.

Animal-based foods are excellent providers of important nutrients including collagen, glucosamine, and chondroitin, all of which are crucial for joint integrity. Collagen, found in abundance in animal connective tissues, is a crucial component of cartilage, the protective padding between joints. Including collagen in the diet may aid in the preservation and regeneration of cartilage, thereby relieving joint pain and stiffness.

The lack of anti-nutrients present in many plant foods, which may lead to inflammation, is a characteristic element of the carnivore diet. By limiting inflammation, elders may have less swelling and stiffness in their joints. This anti-inflammatory action is vital for preserving joint function and reducing the advancement of disorders like arthritis.

Enhanced Cognitive Function: Cognitive decline is a significant issue among seniors, with illnesses like dementia and Alzheimer's growing more prevalent as people age. The carnivore diet, with its concentration on nutrient-dense animal items, may significantly improve cognitive performance.

Omega-3 fatty acids, plentiful in fatty fish and grass-fed meats, play a critical role in brain function. These fatty acids, notably docosahexaenoic acid (DHA), are key components of brain cell membranes and are related to increased cognitive performance. Including enough quantities of omega-3s in the diet may lead to enhanced memory, attention, and general cognitive function for seniors.

The carnivore diet excludes possible inflammatory triggers present in certain plant-based meals. Chronic inflammation has been related to cognitive loss, and by decreasing its prevalence, seniors may have higher cognitive resilience over time.

Managing Chronic Conditions: Seniors commonly battle with chronic diseases such as diabetes, cardiovascular difficulties, and metabolic syndrome. The carnivore diet, with its concentration on animal products and limited carbs, maybe a helpful aid in controlling these disorders.

By eliminating carbs, the diet helps manage blood sugar levels, giving a viable option for seniors coping with diabetes or insulin resistance. This low-carb diet may also aid in weight control, a vital element in avoiding or treating cardiovascular diseases.

The carnivore diet has shown potential in boosting metabolic health. Research shows that it may lead to beneficial changes in lipid profiles, with increasing levels of HDL cholesterol (the "good" cholesterol) and lower levels of triglycerides.

These improvements are suggestive of a decreased risk of cardiovascular disease, an important worry for many elderly. the carnivore diet is an appealing choice for seniors wanting to increase their overall health. Improved joint health, increased cognitive function, and successful treatment of chronic illnesses are key results that may contribute to a more happy and active lifestyle throughout the golden years. As with any dietary adjustment, speaking with healthcare specialists is vital to ensure that individual requirements and health issues are recognized. With the correct supervision, elders may begin on a path toward a healthier and more vibrant future via the power of the carnivorous diet.

CHAPTER FIVE

Navigating the Carnivore Journey

Embarking on a carnivore diet may be a transforming experience for those seeking a drastic adjustment in their eating habits and general well-being. This article attempts to help newcomers through the process of migrating to a carnivore diet, discussing frequent obstacles experienced throughout this trip and proposing practical solutions to guarantee a seamless adaptation.

Transitioning to a Carnivore Diet

The move to a carnivore diet is a change from a typical mixed diet, inclusive of both plant and animal-based meals, to one that largely consists of animal products. Understanding the basics of the carnivorous diet is vital for a successful transition.

The cornerstone of a carnivore diet consists of the intake of animal-sourced foods, including meat, fish, eggs, and dairy. These meals include critical elements such as protein, healthy fats, vitamins, and minerals, which are crucial for nourishing the body.

Eliminating or drastically limiting plant-based foods, including grains, fruits, and vegetables, is a distinguishing aspect of the carnivore diet. While this may appear contrary to standard dietary recommendations, proponents believe that a carnivorous approach coincides with our evolutionary past and may lead to many health advantages.

It's crucial for those switching to a carnivore diet to progressively lower the intake of carbs and plant-based meals while increasing the consumption of animal products. This gradual approach may help the digestive system adjust to the changes and prevent any pain associated with an abrupt dietary transition.

Common Challenges and Solutions: Transitioning to a carnivorous diet might offer some problems, both bodily and psychological. Recognizing and resolving these problems is crucial to a successful and sustained adaptation.

Cravings and Psychological Adjustments: Many people are used to the tastes and sensations of a varied variety of meals. The move to a diet predominantly based on animal products could first induce desires for familiar sensations. To counteract this, it's vital to explore different types of meat, cooking techniques, and seasoning alternatives to enrich the sensory experience of the carnivore diet.

knowing the psychological components of eating and the relevance of mentality in this shift is vital. Framing the move as a good decision for health rather than a restricted diet might lead to a more positive mental attitude.

Digestive Changes: The abrupt increase in dietary fats and proteins may occasionally contribute to digestive discomfort, including bloating, gas, or changes in bowel habits. To aid this transition, folks should gradually increase fat consumption, keep hydrated, and consider digestive supplements if required. Including bone broth and organ meats, which are rich in minerals and supportive of digestive health, may also be useful.

Social and Practical Considerations: Adapting to a carnivorous diet may provide issues in social situations or while eating out. Communicating dietary preferences with friends and family and selecting places that provide carnivore-friendly alternatives may assist navigate these situations. Planning and preparing meals ahead of time can aid in an easier transition, ensuring that adequate food selections are readily accessible.

Nutrient Variability: While animal products offer a vast variety of nutrients, maintaining nutritional diversity is vital for a well-rounded diet. Including a range of meats, organs, and, if permitted, dairy and eggs, helps guarantee a diversified nutritional profile. Consulting with healthcare specialists and selecting suitable supplements may also address particular nutritional problems. Switching to a carnivorous diet is a personal process that takes a mix of knowledge, adaption, and persistence. By knowing the principles of the diet, identifying typical problems, and applying practical solutions, people may traverse this transforming journey with confidence. As with any large dietary change, contact with healthcare specialists is essential to verify that individual nutritional requirements are satisfied and any health risks are addressed. With strategic preparation and dedication to well-being, the carnivore journey may open the door to increased health and vigor.

CHAPTER SIX

Building a Balanced Carnivore Plate for Optimal Health

The carnivore diet, with its concentration on animal products, provides a unique approach to nutrition that may be both transforming and health-promoting. Building a balanced carnivore meal needs careful consideration of protein sources and the integration of healthy fats. In this article, we will discuss the art of designing a well-balanced carnivore plate to provide optimum nutrition for anyone adopting this culinary choice.

Selecting the Right Protein Sources: Proteins are the building blocks of life, and their importance is enhanced on a carnivorous diet. Choosing the correct protein sources is crucial for a balanced meal that satisfies nutritional demands.

Variety in Meat Selection: Diversifying the kinds of meat ingested is vital to guarantee a wide range of nutrients. Opt for a variety of red meats, chicken, fish, and other seafood to supply important amino acids, vitamins, and minerals. Red meats, such as beef and lamb, are especially rich in minerals like iron and zinc, while fatty fish like salmon and mackerel supply omega-3 fatty acids, encouraging heart and brain health.

Inclusion of Organ Meats: Organ meats are nutritious powerhouses, giving a concentrated dose of vitamins and minerals. The liver, for instance, is extremely rich in vitamin A, B vitamins, and iron. Including organ meats in your carnivore dish gives a nutritious punch that compliments the protein supply from muscle meats. While some may find the flavor of organ meats an acquired pleasure, their nutritional advantages make them a desirable supplement to a balanced carnivore diet.

Quality Matters: Opting for high-quality, pasture-raised, and grass-fed beef is vital. These sources often offer a more favorable dietary profile, with greater quantities of omega-3 fatty acids and important vitamins. Quality meat not only boosts the nutritional value of your dish but also promotes ethical and sustainable production methods.

Consideration of Personal Tolerance: Every person reacts differently to various sorts of meat. Some may thrive on a diet strong in beef, while others may enjoy a combination of chicken and fish. Observing how your body responds to various protein sources and changing your plate appropriately gives a tailored and optimum nutritional experience.

Incorporating Healthy Fats: Fats are a cornerstone of the carnivorous diet, providing sustained energy and supporting many biological processes. The idea is to consume healthy fats that help with general well-being.

Embracing Animal Fats: Animal fats, notably those included in meat, chicken skin, and fatty fish, are vital to a balanced carnivore plate. These lipids are high in saturated and monounsaturated fats, needed for hormone synthesis, cell structure, and general metabolic health. While it's vital to appreciate the fat content existing in the selected meats, some persons additionally use extra sources like tallow, lard, or duck fat for cooking and taste improvement.

Including Nutrient-Dense Fats: Beyond animal fats, including nutrient-dense fats from sources like avocados and olives adds diversity to the dish. Avocados, for instance, include monounsaturated fats, fiber, and an assortment of vitamins and minerals. Including these plant-based lipids may contribute to a more well-rounded nutritional profile and boost the overall palatability of the carnivore dish.

Minding Omega-3 to Omega-6 Ratio: Striking a balance between omega-3 and omega-6 fatty acids is vital for sustaining an anti-inflammatory state in the body. While animal fats are often higher in saturated fats, concentrating on fatty fish or supplementing with fish oil may help create a more favorable omega-3 to omega-6 ratio. This balance is related to enhanced cardiovascular health and general inflammation control.

Hydration and Electrolytes: Adequate hydration is crucial on a carnivore diet, particularly given the possible diuretic impact of greater protein consumption. Adding electrolytes, such as salt, potassium, and magnesium, to your diet or via supplementation provides adequate fluid balance and supports normal biological processes.

Creating a balanced carnivore plate is an art that entails a meticulous selection of protein sources and the addition of healthy fats. A broad assortment of meats, inclusion of organ meats, selecting high-quality sources, and embracing both animal and plant-based fats add to a dish that is not only nutritionally strong but also palatably pleasing. As with any dietary strategy, individual tastes and tolerances should be addressed, and engaging with healthcare specialists may give individualized recommendations for the best health on a carnivore diet. With attention to detail and a dedication to nutritional perfection, crafting a balanced carnivore plate becomes a cornerstone for anyone looking to flourish on this unique and revolutionary culinary path.

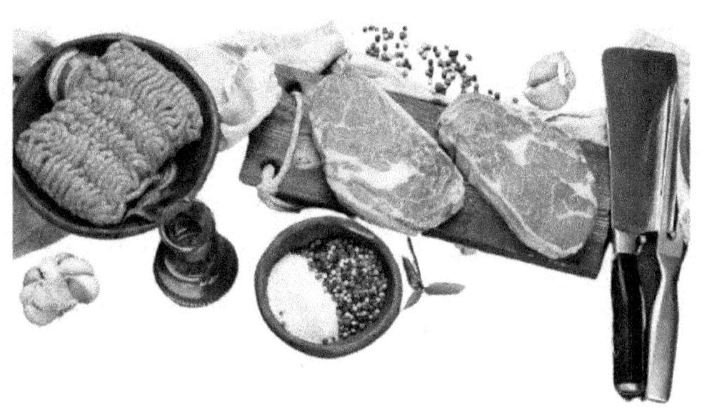

CHAPTER SEVEN

Recipes

10 Irresistible Carnivore Breakfast Recipes for Seniors

Breakfast is the cornerstone of a lively day, and for seniors enjoying the carnivorous lifestyle, it's a chance to launch their morning with tasty and nutrient-packed meals. In this article, we'll examine 10 scrumptious carnivorous breakfast dishes made exclusively for seniors, emphasizing the ingredients and preparation techniques that make each one a delightful and health-promoting option.

Classic Bacon and Eggs

Ingredients:

- ✓ 2 pieces of thick-cut bacon
- ✓ 2 big eggs

Preparation:

- Cook the bacon until crispy in a pan. Remove and cook the eggs in the bacon grease until desired doneness. Serve together for a traditional and protein-rich breakfast.

Smoked Salmon Roll-ups

Ingredients:

- ✓ 4 ounces smoked salmon
- ✓ 2 ounces cream cheese
- ✓ Chives (optional)

Preparation:

- Spread cream cheese over smoked salmon pieces, wrap them up, and fasten with chives if desired. A wonderful and omega-3-rich breakfast alternative.

Egg and Sausage Muffins

Ingredients:

- ✓ 4 big eggs
- ✓ 8 breakfast sausages (sugar-free)
- ✓ Salt and pepper to taste

Preparation:

- Whisk eggs, season, and pour into a muffin tray. Add a sausage to each cup and bake until the eggs are set. A handy and protein-packed breakfast.

Steak and Avocado Salad

Ingredients:

- ✓ 6 ounces leftover steak, sliced 1 ripe avocado, sliced
- ✓ Salt and pepper to taste

Preparation:

- Combine cut steak and avocado, and season to taste. A full and fulfilling breakfast that delivers important nutrients.

Egg and Cheese Breakfast Casserole

Ingredients:

- ✓ 6 big eggs
- ✓ 1 cup shredded cheddar cheese
- ✓ Salt and pepper to taste

Preparation:

- Whisk eggs, season, then add in shredded cheese. Bake until set for a tasty and protein-rich breakfast dish.

Chicken Liver Pâté

Ingredients:

- ✓ 1 pound chicken livers
- ✓ 1/2 cup butter
- ✓ Salt and pepper to taste

Preparation:

- Sauté chicken livers in butter, then mix until smooth. Refrigerate and serve as a spread for a nutrient-dense breakfast.

Sausage and Egg Breakfast Skillet

Ingredients:

- ✓ 8 ounces ground breakfast sausage
- ✓ 4 big eggs
- ✓ Salt and pepper to taste

Preparation:

Cook sausage in a pan, add whisked eggs, and scramble together. A quick and tasty one-pan breakfast.

Baked Ham and Cheese Omelet

Ingredients:

- ✓ 6 big eggs
- ✓ 1 cup diced ham
- ✓ 1/2 cup shredded Swiss cheese

Preparation:

- Whisk eggs, add ham and cheese, and bake until eggs are set. A delicious and protein-packed omelet.

Ground Beef Breakfast Bowl

Ingredients:

- ✓ 8 ounces ground beef
- ✓ 2 eggs
- ✓ Salt and pepper to taste

Preparation:

- Cook ground beef, season, then top with fried eggs. A substantial and delicious breakfast dish.

Turkey and Cheese Roll-ups

Ingredients:

- ✓ 6 slices turkey
- ✓ 6 slices cheddar cheese
- ✓ Mustard for dipping (optional)

Preparation:

- Layer turkey slices with cheddar cheese, wrap them up and serve with mustard if preferred. An easy and tasty breakfast choice.

These 10 carnivore breakfast dishes for seniors give a delectable selection of alternatives to jumpstart their day with nutrient-dense, protein-rich meals. From conventional bacon and eggs to innovative steak and avocado salads, these dishes appeal to various preferences while ensuring seniors obtain the critical nutrients they need for optimum health. With careful attention to ingredients and preparation techniques, these breakfast alternatives give a pleasurable and health-promoting start to each day.

10 Carnivore Diet Lunch Recipes Tailored for Seniors

As seniors begin on their golden years, the necessity of a nutrient-rich diet cannot be stressed. The carnivore diet, defined by the intake of animal products, has promise in satisfying the special nutritional demands of seniors. This post includes 10 particular carnivore diet lunch dishes, intended to not only accommodate the unique dietary needs of seniors but also to thrill their palates with tasty and fulfilling meals.

Recipe 1: Chicken Caesar Salad

Ingredients:

- ✓ 1 pound grilled chicken breast, sliced Romaine lettuce, chopped 1/4 cup grated Parmesan cheese
- ✓ Caesar dressing (olive oil, anchovies, garlic, Dijon mustard)
- ✓ To taste, season with salt and pepper

Preparation:

- ✓ Combine grilled chicken, chopped romaine lettuce, and Parmesan cheese in a bowl.
- ✓ Drizzle with Caesar dressing.
- ✓ Toss gently and season with salt and pepper.

Recipe 2: Egg Salad Lettuce Wraps

Parts and pieces:

- ✓ 6 hard-boiled eggs, chopped
- ✓ 1/4 cup mayonnaise
- ✓ Dijon mustard to taste
- ✓ Iceberg lettuce leaves
- ✓ To taste, season with salt and pepper

Preparation:

- Mix chopped eggs with mayonnaise and Dijon mustard.
- Spoon the egg mixture over individual lettuce leaves.
- Season with salt and pepper.

Recipe 3: Tuna Avocado Boats

Ingredients:

- ✓ 2 cans of tuna, drained 2 ripe avocados, halved 1/4 cup chopped celery
- ✓ Olive oil, lemon juice, salt, and pepper to taste

Preparation:

- In a bowl, add tuna and sliced celery.
- Drizzle with olive oil and lemon juice.
- Spoon the tuna mixture into avocado halves.
- Season with salt and pepper.

Recipe 4: Beef and Spinach Omelet

Parts and pieces:

- ✓ 4 big eggs
- ✓ 1/2 pound ground beef
- ✓ Handful of fresh spinach, chopped
- ✓ To taste, season with salt and pepper

Preparation:

- ✓ Brown ground beef in a pan over medium heat.
- ✓ In a bowl, beat eggs and add chopped spinach.
- ✓ Pour the egg and spinach mixture over the meat.
- ✓ Cook until the eggs are set, then fold in half.

Recipe 5: Lamb Kebabs with Mint Yogurt Sauce

Parts and pieces:

- ✓ 1 pound lamb cubes
- ✓ Olive oil
- ✓ Fresh mint leaves, chopped 1 cup plain Greek yogurt
- ✓ To taste, season with salt and pepper

Preparation:

- Thread lamb chunks onto skewers and drizzle with olive oil.
- Grill until cooked to the desired doneness.
- Mix chopped mint with Greek yogurt for a dipping sauce.
- Season meat with salt and pepper and serve with the mint yogurt sauce.

Recipe 6: Bacon-wrapped Asparagus Bundles

Ingredients:

- ✓ Fresh asparagus spears
- ✓ Bacon slices
- ✓ Olive oil
- ✓ Salt and pepper to taste

Preparation:

- Preheat the oven to 400°F (200°C).
- Wrap a piece of bacon around several asparagus shoots to make bundles.
- Place the bundles on a baking sheet, sprinkle with olive oil, and season with salt and pepper.
- Bake until the bacon is crispy.

Recipe 7: Turkey and Cheese Roll-ups

Parts and pieces:

- ✓ Deli-sliced turkey
- ✓ Sliced cheese (cheddar, Swiss, or your pick)
- ✓ Mustard for spreading

- Pickle spears

Preparation:

- Lay out turkey slices and add a piece of cheese to each.
- Spread mustard on the cheese.
- Roll up the turkey and cheese to make roll-ups.
- Serve with pickle spears on the side.

Recipe 8: Pork Carnitas Lettuce Wraps

Parts and pieces:

- ✓ 1 pound pork shoulder, shredded Iceberg lettuce leaves
- ✓ Diced tomatoes, onions, and cilantro for topping
- ✓ Lime wedges
- ✓ To taste, season with salt and pepper

Preparation:

- Season pork shoulder with salt and pepper and slow-cook until tender.
- Spoon shredded pork onto lettuce leaves.
- Top with diced tomatoes, onions, and cilantro.

- Squeeze lime wedges over the top.

Recipe 9: Grilled Sardines with Lemon

Ingredients:

- ✓ Fresh sardines, cleaned Olive oil
- ✓ Lemon slices
- ✓ To taste, season with salt and pepper

Preparation:

- Brush sardines with olive oil and season with salt and pepper.
- Grill till cooked through.
- Serve with lemon slices for a pleasant accent.

Recipe 10: Salmon Patties

Ingredients:

- ✓ 1 pound canned salmon, drained 2 eggs
- ✓ Almond flour
- ✓ Diced green onions
- ✓ To taste, season with salt and pepper

- In a bowl, mix drained salmon, beaten eggs, almond flour, and green onions.
- Form the mixture into patties.
- Pan-fry until golden brown on both sides.

These 10 carnivore diet lunch ideas have been thoughtfully developed to supply seniors with not only the vital nutrients needed for their well-being but also with a diversity of tastes and textures to make their meals interesting and gratifying. Embracing the carnivore lifestyle may be a delightful and beneficial decision for seniors, provided they acquire the nourishment essential to flourish in their golden years.

10 Satisfying Carnivore Diet Dinner Recipes

As seniors traverse the golden hours of their day, the value of a nutrient-dense meal cannot be stressed. The carnivore diet, focused on animal products, is a viable path for seniors to maintain maximum health. In this article, we look into 10 particular carnivore diet supper dishes customized to the unique nutritional demands of seniors, giving both sustenance and gourmet enjoyment.

Recipe 1: Ribeye Steak with Garlic Butter

Ingredients:

- ✓ 2 ribeye steaks
- ✓ 4 tbsp grass-fed butter
- ✓ 4 cloves garlic, minced
- ✓ To taste, season with salt and pepper

Preparation:

- Season ribeye steaks with salt and pepper.
- Grill or pan-sear the steaks to the desired doneness.
- In a saucepan, heat butter and sauté minced garlic.
- Pour garlic butter over the steaks before serving.

Recipe 2: Chicken Thighs with Lemon and Herbs

Parts and pieces:

- ✓ 4 bone-in, skin-on chicken thighs
- ✓ Zest and juice of 1 lemon
- ✓ Fresh thyme and rosemary
- ✓ To taste, season with salt and pepper

Preparation:

- Preheat the oven to 375°F (190°C).
- Season chicken thighs with lemon zest, lemon juice, thyme, rosemary, salt, and pepper.
- Roast in the oven until the skin is crispy and the internal temperature reaches 165°F (74°C).

Recipe 3: Seared Scallops with Garlic Ghee

Parts and pieces:

- ✓ 1 pound fresh scallops
- ✓ 2 tbsp ghee
- ✓ 3 cloves garlic, minced

✓ Fresh parsley for garnish

✓ To taste, season with salt and pepper

Preparation:

- Pat scallops dry and season with salt and pepper.

- Heat ghee in a pan over medium-high heat.

- Sear scallops for 2-3 minutes on each side or until golden brown.

- Sprinkle minced garlic over the scallops and sprinkle with fresh parsley before serving.

Recipe 4: Pork Ribs with Dry Rub

Parts and pieces:

✓ 2 racks of pork ribs

✓ Dry rub (paprika, garlic powder, onion powder, salt, pepper)

✓ Sugar-free barbecue sauce (optional)

Preparation:

- Preheat the oven to 275°F (135°C).

- Rub the pork ribs with the dry rub, covering both sides.

- Bake in the oven for 3-4 hours until soft.

- Optionally, brush with sugar-free barbecue sauce before serving.

Recipe 5: Lamb Shank Stew

Ingredients:

- ✓ 2 lamb shanks
- ✓ 1 onion, diced 2 carrots, sliced 2 celery stalks, chopped Beef broth
- ✓ To taste, season with salt and pepper

Preparation:

- Brown lamb shanks in a saucepan over medium heat.
- Add diced onion, sliced carrots, and chopped celery.
- Pour in enough beef broth to cover the items.
- Simmer for 2-3 hours until the meat is cooked.

Recipe 6: Grilled Swordfish Steaks

Ingredients:

- ✓ 2 swordfish steaks
- ✓ Olive oil
- ✓ Lemon juice

- ✓ Fresh dill for garnish
- ✓ To taste, season with salt and pepper

Preparation:

- Brush swordfish steaks with olive oil and season with salt and pepper.
- Grill for 4-5 minutes on each side or until cooked through.
- Drizzle with lemon juice and garnish with fresh dill before serving.

Recipe 7: Ground Beef and Eggplant Casserole

Ingredients:

- ✓ 1 pound ground beef
- ✓ 2 medium eggplants, sliced Tomato sauce
- ✓ Grated Parmesan cheese
- ✓ To taste, season with salt and pepper

Preparation:

- Brown ground beef in a pan over medium heat.
- Layer sliced eggplants in a baking dish.

- Top with ground meat, tomato sauce, and Parmesan cheese.
- Bake in the oven at 375°F (190°C) for 30-40 minutes or until bubbling.

Recipe 8: Turkey Bacon-wrapped Brussels Sprouts

Parts and pieces:

- ✓ Brussels sprouts Turkey bacon slices
- ✓ Olive oil
- ✓ To taste, season with salt and pepper

Preparation:

- Preheat the oven to 400°F (200°C).
- Wrap each Brussels sprout with a piece of turkey bacon.
- Place on a baking sheet, sprinkle with olive oil, and season with salt and pepper.
- Bake until the bacon is crispy.

Recipe 9: Bison Burger Lettuce Wraps

Ingredients:

- ✓ 1-pound ground bison
- ✓ Lettuce leaves
- ✓ Sliced tomatoes, onions, and pickles for topping
- ✓ Mustard and mayonnaise for dressing
- ✓ To taste, season with salt and pepper

Preparation:

- Form ground bison into burger patties and season with salt and pepper.
- Grill or pan-cook until thoroughly done.
- Place each bison burger in a lettuce leaf.
- Top with sliced tomatoes, onions, pickles, mustard, and mayonnaise.

Recipe 10: Salmon and Avocado Salad

Parts and pieces:

- ✓ 2 salmon fillets, grilled and flakes
- ✓ Mixed salad greens
- ✓ 1 avocado, diced Olive oil, and lemon juice for dressing

✓ To taste, season with salt and pepper

Preparation:

- Combine grilled salmon, mixed salad leaves, and cubed avocado in a bowl.
- Drizzle with olive oil and lemon juice.
- Toss gently and season with salt and pepper.

In adopting these 10 carnivore diet supper recipes, seniors may enjoy in a range of tasty and gratifying foods that cater precisely to their nutritional requirements. These dishes not only offer a healthy intake of critical nutrients but also promise a pleasurable culinary experience, making the carnivore diet a savory and nutritious option for seniors for their evening meals.

10 Carnivore Diet Seafood Recipes for Seniors

As elders navigate the seas of aging, the significance of a nutrient-rich diet becomes crucial. The carnivore diet, concentrated upon animal products, maybe a beacon of health for seniors, particularly when complemented with the treasures of the sea. This article goes into 10 particular carnivore diet seafood dishes meant to cater to the unique nutritional demands of seniors, delivering not only tasty and flavorful alternatives but also a treasure trove of necessary elements.

Recipe 1: Grilled Lemon Garlic Shrimp

Ingredients:

- ✓ 1 lb big shrimp, peeled and deveined
- ✓ 2 tbsp olive oil
- ✓ Zest and juice of 1 lemon
- ✓ 3 cloves garlic, minced
- ✓ To taste, season with salt and pepper

Preparation:

- In a bowl, combine shrimp with olive oil, lemon zest, lemon juice, chopped garlic, salt, and pepper.
- Thread shrimp onto skewers and cook for 2-3 minutes on each side.

Recipe 2: Baked Lemon Dill Salmon

Parts and pieces:

- ✓ 2 salmon fillets

- ✓ 2 tbsp melted butter

- ✓ Zest and juice of 1 lemon

- ✓ Fresh dill

- ✓ To taste, season with salt and pepper

Preparation:

- • Preheat the oven to 375°F (190°C).

- • Place salmon fillets on a baking sheet.

- • Mix melted butter with lemon zest, lemon juice, fresh dill, salt, and pepper.

- • Brush the mixture over the salmon and bake for 15-20 minutes or until the fish flakes easily.

Recipe 3: Garlic Butter Lobster Tails

Ingredients:

- ✓ 4 lobster tails

- ✓ 1/2 cup melted butter

- ✓ 4 cloves garlic, minced

- ✓ Fresh parsley for garnish

- ✓ To taste, season with salt and pepper

Preparation:

- ✓ Preheat the oven to 425°F (220°C).

✓ Cut the top of each lobster tail lengthwise.

✓ Mix melted butter with minced garlic, salt, and pepper.

✓ Brush the lobster tails with the garlic butter mixture and bake for 15-20 minutes.

✓ Garnish with fresh parsley before serving.

Recipe 4: Tuna Steak with Sesame Crust

Parts and pieces:

✓ 2 tuna steaks

✓ 2 tbsp sesame seeds

✓ 2 tbsp soy sauce

✓ 1 tbsp sesame oil

✓ To taste, season with salt and pepper

Preparation:

• Season tuna steaks with salt and pepper.

• Coat each steak with sesame seeds, pressing them into the surface.

• In a pan, heat sesame oil over medium-high heat.

• Sear tuna steaks for 1-2 minutes on each side.

• Drizzle with soy sauce before serving.

Recipe 5: Coconut Lime Shrimp Skewers

Ingredients:

- ✓ 1 lb big shrimp, peeled and deveined
- ✓ 1/2 cup coconut milk
- ✓ Zest and juice of 2 limes
- ✓ 2 tbsp chopped cilantro
- ✓ To taste, season with salt and pepper

Preparation:

- In a bowl, add coconut milk, lime zest, lime juice, chopped cilantro, salt, and pepper.
- Thread shrimp onto skewers and marinate in the coconut lime salsa for 30 minutes.
- Grill shrimp skewers for 2-3 minutes on each side.

Recipe 6: Scallops with Bacon and Rosemary

Parts and pieces:

- ✓ 1 pound fresh scallops
- ✓ Bacon slices
- ✓ Fresh rosemary sprigs

✓ To taste, season with salt and pepper

Preparation:

- Wrap each scallop with a piece of bacon and fasten with a toothpick.
- Season with salt and pepper and lay a rosemary leaf on top.
- Grill or pan-sear until the bacon is crispy.

Recipe 7: Lemon Butter Cod Fish

Parts and pieces:

✓ 4 cod fillets

✓ 4 tbsp grass-fed butter

✓ Zest and juice of 1 lemon

✓ Fresh parsley for garnish

✓ To taste, season with salt and pepper

Preparation:

- Preheat the oven to 400°F (200°C).
- Place fish fillets on a baking sheet.
- Mix melted butter with lemon zest, lemon juice, salt, and pepper.

- Brush the mixture over the fish and bake for 15-20 minutes.
- Garnish with fresh parsley before serving.

Recipe 8: Garlic Herb Grilled Squid

Parts and pieces:

- ✓ 1-pound squid tubes, cleaned and scored
- ✓ 3 tbsp olive oil
- ✓ Fresh herbs (rosemary, thyme, oregano)
- ✓ 4 cloves garlic, minced
- ✓ Salt and pepper to taste

Preparation:

- In a bowl, combine olive oil, fresh herbs, minced garlic, salt, and pepper.
- Marinate squid tubes in the marinade for at least 30 minutes.
- Grill squid tubes for 2-3 minutes on each side.

Recipe 9: Cajun Shrimp and Sausage Skillet

Parts and pieces:

- ✓ 1 lb big shrimp, peeled and deveined
- ✓ 1 pound smoked sausage, sliced Cajun seasoning
- ✓ 2 tbsp olive oil
- ✓ To taste, season with salt and pepper

Preparation:

- In a pan, heat olive oil over medium-high heat.
- Add sliced sausage and heat until browned.
- Add shrimp and sprinkle with Cajun spice.
- Cook for 2-3 minutes until shrimp are pink and cooked through.

Recipe 10: Crab Stuffed Avocado

Parts and pieces:

- ✓ 1 pound lump crab meat
- ✓ 2 avocados, halved
- ✓ 2 tbsp mayonnaise
- ✓ 1 tbsp Dijon mustard

- ✓ Fresh chives for garnish
- ✓ To taste, season with salt and pepper

Preparation:

- In a bowl, mix lump crab meat, mayonnaise, Dijon mustard, salt, and pepper.
- Spoon the crab mixture into half avocados.
- Garnish with fresh chives before serving.

These 10 seafood dishes for the carnivore diet have been meticulously created to give seniors with a tasty and nutrient-rich eating experience. From luscious shrimp and tasty salmon to delicate scallops and strong lobster, these dishes guarantee seniors can relish the ocean's delights while prioritizing their health. The carnivorous diet, packed with seafood pleasures, becomes a gustatory voyage that not only satisfies the palette but also improves the well-being of seniors throughout their golden years.

10 Carnivore Diet Snack Recipes for Seniors

In the quest for healthy aging, the carnivore diet appears as a potential option for seniors, concentrating on nutrient-dense animal products. While the major meals play a critical role, snacks may bring diversity and enjoyment to a senior's daily diet. This article covers 10 particular carnivore diet snack foods customized to the nutritional requirements of seniors, delivering tasty, easy-to-prepare solutions that guarantee both flavor and health are emphasized.

Recipe 1: Deviled Eggs with Bacon

Ingredients:

- ✓ 6 hard-boiled eggs, halved
- ✓ 3 tbsp mayonnaise
- ✓ 2 tsp Dijon mustard
- ✓ To taste, season with salt and pepper
- ✓ Cooked bacon pieces for topping

- Scoop out the egg yolks and combine with mayonnaise, Dijon mustard, salt, and pepper.
- Spoon the mixture back into the egg white halves.
- Top each deviled egg with bacon pieces.

Recipe 2: Parmesan Crisps

Ingredients:

- ✓ 1 cup grated Parmesan cheese

Preparation:

- Preheat the oven to 375°F (190°C).
- Line a baking sheet with parchment paper.
- Spoon tiny mounds of grated Parmesan onto the sheet.
- Bake for 5-7 minutes or until golden brown and crispy.

Recipe 3: Beef Jerky

Ingredients:

- ✓ 1 lb lean beef, thinly sliced Marinade (soy sauce, Worcestershire sauce, garlic powder, onion powder, black pepper)

Preparation:

- Mix the marinade ingredients in a bowl.
- Coat the beef slices in the marinade and let rest for at least 2 hours.
- Dehydrate the marinated beef slices until thoroughly dry.

Recipe 4: Chicken Liver Pops

Parts and pieces:

- ✓ Chicken livers Bacon slices
- ✓ Toothpicks

Preparation:

- Wrap each chicken liver with a bacon slice and fasten with a toothpick.

- Bake in the oven at 400°F (200°C) until the bacon is crispy.

Recipe 5: Smoked Salmon Roll-ups

Parts and pieces:

- ✓ Smoked salmon slices
- ✓ Cream cheese
- ✓ Chives

Preparation:

- ✓ Spread cream cheese atop smoked salmon pieces.
- ✓ Roll the pieces and fasten them with chives.

Recipe 6: Sardine Stuffed Avocado

Ingredients:

- ✓ Canned sardines
- ✓ Avocados, halved and pitted Lemon juice
- ✓ To taste, season with salt and pepper

Preparation:

- Mix tinned sardines with lemon juice, salt, and pepper.

- Spoon the sardine mixture into half avocados.

Recipe 7: Cheese and Pepperoni Bites

Ingredients:

- ✓ Sliced pepperoni
- ✓ Sliced cheese (cheddar, mozzarella, or your pick)

Preparation:

- Place a piece of cheese on a slice of pepperoni.
- Fold or fold the pepperoni around the cheese.

Recipe 8: Ham and Cream Cheese Rolls

Ingredients:

- ✓ Sliced deli ham Cream cheese Dijon mustard

Preparation:

- Spread cream cheese and Dijon mustard on a piece of deli ham.
- Roll the ham into a tight cylinder.

Recipe 9: Bacon-wrapped Shrimp

Parts and pieces:

- ✓ Large shrimp, peeled and deveined Bacon slices

Preparation:

- Wrap each shrimp with a piece of bacon.
- Secure with toothpicks.
- Grill or bake until the bacon is crispy.

Recipe 10: Prosciutto-wrapped Asparagus

Parts and pieces:

Fresh asparagus spears

Prosciutto slices

Olive oil

Salt and pepper to taste

Preparation:

- Wrap each asparagus spear with a piece of prosciutto.
- Drizzle with olive oil and season with salt and pepper.

- Bake in the oven at 400°F (200°C) until asparagus is tender.

These 10 carnivore diet snack dishes provide seniors with a tempting selection of alternatives that not only please their taste buds but also correspond with the concepts of a nutrient-dense carnivore diet. From protein-packed deviled eggs to savory Parmesan crisps and decadent bacon-wrapped shrimp, these snacks contribute to the overall well-being of seniors by ensuring they acquire critical nutrients while enjoying delectable and gratifying morsels between meals.

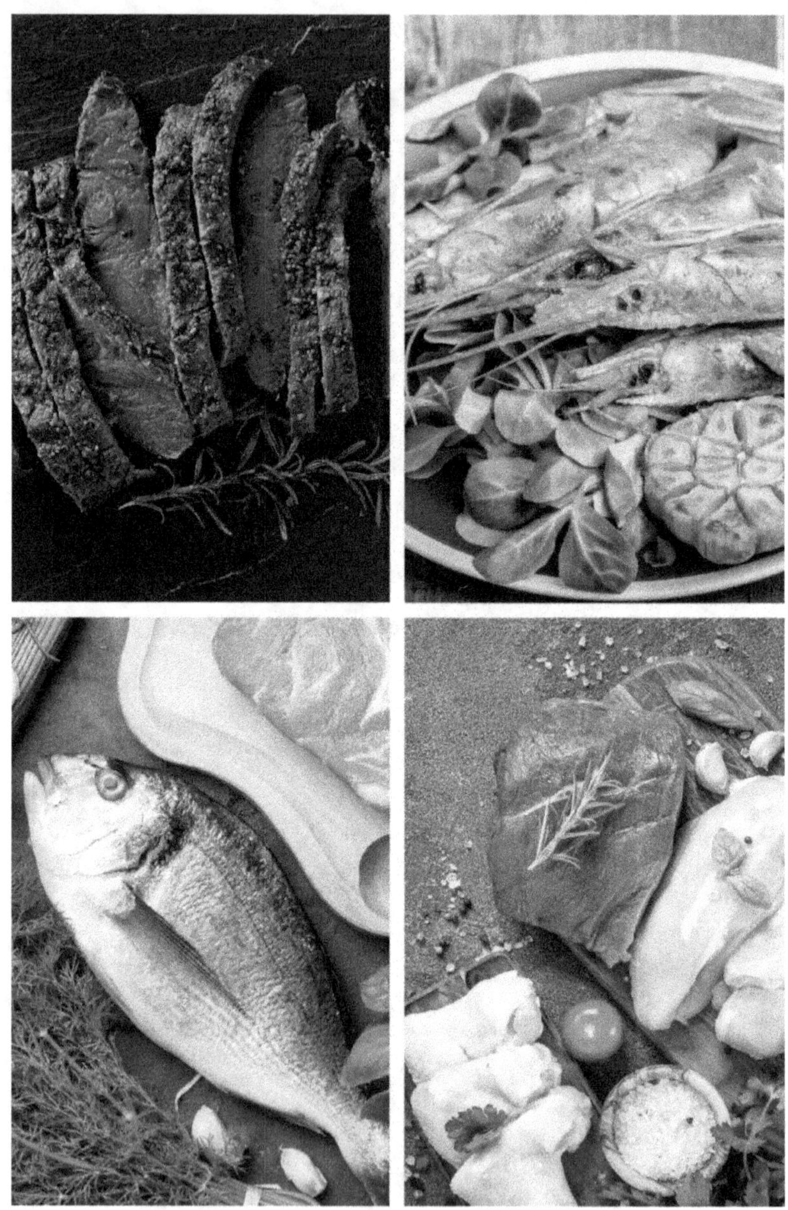

CHAPTER EIGHT

28-day meal plan

Creating a thorough 28-day meal plan for the Carnivore Diet for seniors takes careful consideration of nutritional demands, variety, and taste. The diet below contains a combination of meat, fish, eggs, and some dairy, ensuring seniors acquire critical nutrients while enjoying a broad selection of meals.

Day 1:

Breakfast: Scrambled Eggs with Ground Beef

Lunch: Grilled Salmon Salad with Avocado

Dinner: Ribeye Steak with Garlic Butter

Snack: Parmesan Crisps

Day 2:

Breakfast: Bacon and Eggs

Lunch: Chicken Caesar Salad

Dinner: Tuna Steak with Sesame Crust

Snack: Beef Jerky

Day 3:

Breakfast: Sardine Stuffed Avocado

Lunch: Pork Ribs with Dry Rub

Dinner: Coconut Lime Shrimp Skewers

Snack: Prosciutto-wrapped Asparagus

Day 4:

Breakfast: Deviled Eggs with Bacon

Lunch: Beef and Broccoli Stir-Fry

Dinner: Garlic Butter Lobster Tails

Snack: Cheese and Pepperoni Bites

Day 5:

Breakfast: Chicken Liver Pops

Lunch: Turkey Bacon-wrapped Brussels Sprouts

Dinner: Smoked Salmon Roll-ups

Snack: Ham and Cream Cheese Rolls

Day 6:

Breakfast: Grilled Lemon Garlic Shrimp

Lunch: Lamb Chops with Rosemary

Dinner: Bison Burger Lettuce Wraps

Snack: Bacon-wrapped Shrimp

Day 7:

Breakfast: Baked Lemon Dill Salmon

Lunch: Ground Beef and Cabbage Skillet

Dinner: Seared Scallops with Garlic Ghee

Snack: Crab Stuffed Avocado

Day 8:

Breakfast: Parmesan Crisps with Cream Cheese

Lunch: Chicken Thighs with Lemon and Herbs

Dinner: Lemon Butter Cod Fish Snack: Cheese and Sausage Platter

Day 9:

Breakfast: Tuna Avocado Boats

Lunch: Beef Jerky

Dinner: Grilled Swordfish Steaks

Snack: Cheese and Olive Skewers

Day 10:

Breakfast: Scrambled Eggs with Ground Lamb

Lunch: Shrimp and Asparagus Skewers

Dinner: Ground Beef and Eggplant Casserole

Snack: Turkey and Cheese Roll-ups

Day 11:

Breakfast: Bacon and Eggs

Lunch: Cod Fish with Lemon Butter Sauce

Dinner: Pork Carnitas Lettuce Wraps

Snack: Parmesan Crisps

Day 12:

Breakfast: Sardine Stuffed Avocado

Lunch: Beef and Spinach Omelette

Dinner: Chicken Liver Pate Snack: Beef Jerky

Day 13:

Breakfast: Deviled Eggs with Bacon

Lunch: Lamb Kebabs with Mint Yogurt Sauce

Dinner: Shrimp and Cabbage Stir-Fry

Snack: Prosciutto-wrapped Asparagus

Day 14:

Breakfast: Grilled Lemon Garlic Shrimp

Lunch: Bison Stew with Vegetables

Dinner: Salmon Patties

Snack: Cheese and Pepperoni Bites

Day 15:

Breakfast: Chicken Liver Pops

Lunch: Turkey Bacon-wrapped Brussels Sprouts

Dinner: Smoked Salmon Roll-ups

Snack: Cheese and Olive Skewers

Day 16:

Breakfast: Baked Lemon Dill Salmon

Lunch: Ground Beef and Cabbage Skillet

Dinner: Seared Scallops with Garlic Ghee

Snack: Crab Stuffed Avocado

Day 17:

Breakfast: Parmesan Crisps with Cream Cheese

Lunch: Chicken Thighs with Lemon and Herbs

Dinner: Lemon Butter Cod Fish Snack: Cheese and Sausage Platter

Day 18:

Breakfast: Tuna Avocado Boats

Lunch: Beef Jerky

Dinner: Grilled Swordfish Steaks

Snack: Cheese and Olive Skewers

Day 19:

Breakfast: Scrambled Eggs with Ground Lamb

Lunch: Shrimp and Asparagus Skewers

Dinner: Ground Beef and Eggplant Casserole

Snack: Turkey and Cheese Roll-ups

Day 20:

Breakfast: Bacon and Eggs

Lunch: Cod Fish with Lemon Butter Sauce

Dinner: Pork Carnitas Lettuce Wraps

Snack: Parmesan Crisps

Day 21:

Breakfast: Sardine Stuffed Avocado

Lunch: Beef and Spinach Omelet

Dinner: Chicken Liver Pate Snack: Beef Jerky

Day 22:

Breakfast: Deviled Eggs with Bacon

Lunch: Lamb Kebabs with Mint Yogurt Sauce

Dinner: Shrimp and Cabbage Stir-Fry

Snack: Prosciutto-wrapped Asparagus

Day 23:

Breakfast: Grilled Lemon Garlic Shrimp

Lunch: Bison Stew with Vegetables

Dinner: Salmon Patties

Snack: Cheese and Pepperoni Bites

Day 24:

Breakfast: Chicken Liver Pops

Lunch: Turkey Bacon-wrapped Brussels Sprouts

Dinner: Smoked Salmon Roll-ups

Snack: Cheese and Olive Skewers

Day 25:

Breakfast: Baked Lemon Dill Salmon

Lunch: Ground Beef and Cabbage Skillet

Dinner: Seared Scallops with Garlic Ghee

Snack: Crab Stuffed Avocado

Day 26:

Breakfast: Parmesan Crisps with Cream Cheese

Lunch: Chicken Thighs with Lemon and Herbs

Dinner: Lemon Butter Cod Fish Snack: Cheese and Sausage Platter

Day 27:

Breakfast: Tuna Avocado Boats

Lunch: Beef Jerky

Dinner: Grilled Swordfish Steaks

Snack: Cheese and Olive Skewers

Day 28:

Breakfast: Scrambled Eggs with Ground Lamb

Lunch: Shrimp and Asparagus Skewers

Dinner: Ground Beef and Eggplant Casserole

Snack: Turkey and Cheese Roll-ups

This meal plan offers seniors a balanced and diverse carnivore diet, ensuring they acquire critical nutrients and enjoy a delectable choice of meals over 28 days. Always contact with a healthcare practitioner before making large changes to dietary habits, particularly for seniors or persons with certain health issues.

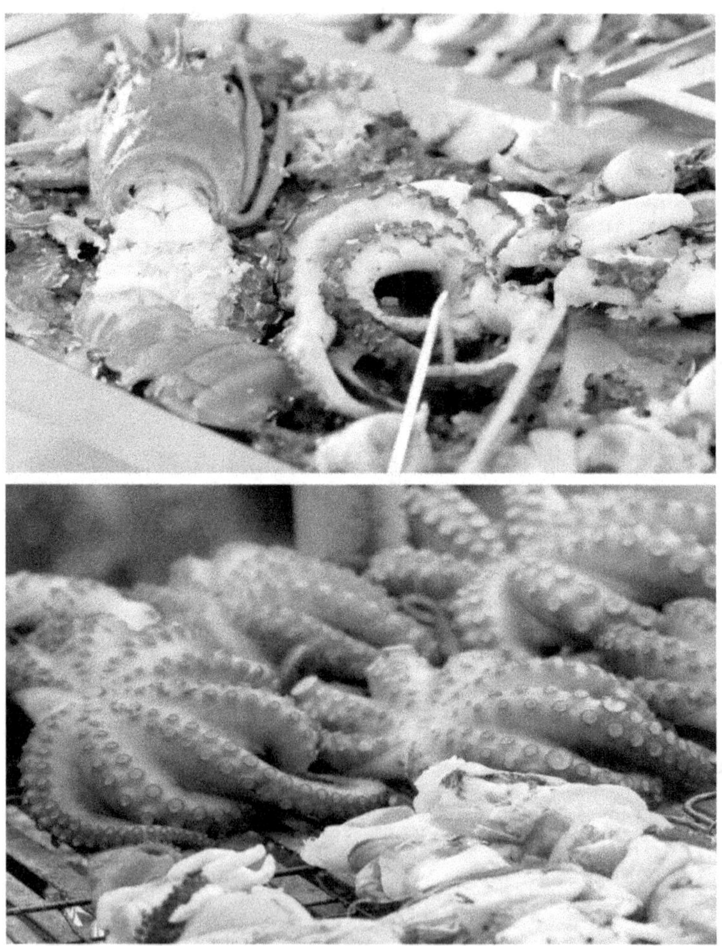

Embracing Vitality in the Golden Years with the Carnivore Diet

As we approach the last chapter of our inquiry into the world of the Carnivore Diet for seniors, it's a suitable occasion to reflect on the transforming adventure we've made together. This culinary voyage has not only uncovered the subtleties of the Carnivore Diet but has also lighted a route toward greater well-being, resilience, and vitality in the golden years.

Highlights from Our Culinary Expedition

Understanding Senior Nutrition: We started our trip by looking into the special nutritional demands of seniors, noting the subtle alterations in metabolism, muscle mass, and digestive processes that characterize this wonderful chapter of life.

The Basics of the Carnivore Diet: Navigating the carnivorous wilderness, we studied the basic concepts of the

Carnivore Diet. From the rejection of plant-based meals to the exaltation of animal fats, each rule was a stepping stone toward a simpler, more primitive approach to eating.

Health Benefits for elders: Throughout our adventure, we revealed the possible health benefits of the Carnivore Diet for elders. From enhanced joint health and cognitive function to successful treatment of chronic illnesses, the diet emerged as a significant ally in supporting general well-being.

Meal Planning and Recipes: The heart of our adventure was in the kitchen, where we found the skill of producing tasty and nutrient-rich meals designed for seniors. From pan-seared fish to grilled ribeye steak, each item was a tribute to the elegance and diversity that the Carnivore Diet can provide.

Addressing Concerns and Misconceptions: We faced the controversy surrounding the Carnivore Diet, meticulously deconstructing the falsehoods and safety implications. By addressing the concerns and giving evidence-based insights, we hoped to enable seniors to make educated decisions about their food choices.

Success Stories and Testimonials: The pages of our book rang with the inspirational experiences of seniors who began on the Carnivore Diet adventure. Real-life experiences showed the possibility for increased energy, enhanced health indicators, and a joy for life that defied conventional assumptions.

The Road Ahead:

As we complete this chapter, it's crucial to remember that the Carnivore Diet is not a one-size-fits-all answer. It's a toolbox, a culinary canvas, encouraging seniors to tailor their approach based on individual requirements, tastes, and health concerns.

In adopting the Carnivore Diet, seniors go on an adventure that surpasses the limitations of standard nutrition. It's a celebration of the basic link between people and the food found in the animal world. Through conscious investigation and an open-hearted acceptance of this dietary philosophy, seniors have the chance to rethink their relationship with food and unleash a chapter of life filled with vigor, sustenance, and pleasure.

May this book serve as a guide, a companion, and a source of inspiration for seniors looking to navigate the Carnivore Diet world. As we say goodbye to these pages, let us take on the knowledge learned, appreciate the flavors found, and, above all, rejoice in the possibility of a lively and joyful trip into the golden years with the Carnivore Diet as a loyal partner.

Good luck in the kitchen!

www.ingramcontent.com/pod-product-compliance
Lightning Source LLC
Chambersburg PA
CBHW050832260726
48660CB00006B/2199